# The Super Weight Loss Diet

## How to lose weight in 30 days

# Table of Contents

# Introduction

There is a story behind everyone who is fighting the weight loss battle. Nobody went to bed thin and woke up overweight.

It could be the result of years of conditioning including how we were raised to associate food with good emotions. As kids, our parents showed love through food. Many of our happy memories are associated with food – memories of the sound the ice cream truck made, family dinners at a local Italian restaurant, or breakfast with friends at the local diner.

It could be because somewhere along the way, we learned to use food as a way to cope with unpleasant emotions like stress...or sadness. It's so easy to turn to food when we have so many deadlines at work, or when we get so tired taking care of the kids.

But this also means one thing: It *is* reversible. There *is* something you can do. And this book will be your blue print on what exactly it is that you can do – from how to approach weight loss to food recommendations to actual food preparation instructions.

There's also a chapter on a specific weight loss technique – intermittent fasting – for those who want a faster way to lose weight and those who could bear a stricter regimen.

But what really makes this book different is that it was created with one thing in mind: quick and sustainable weight loss.

Conventionally, dieting in itself is already hard, so we decided to make dieting something that you would want to get into – and something that you can do for a long time. And the best part is, you don't have to wait long to see the results.

A diet regimen spanning 30 days, when done right, will mean losing 8 pounds (anything more than that is possible but could be harmful). With that degree of weight loss, you will already see a big difference not just in your waistline but also in the way you perform day to day activities.

- You'll see that you have more energy to do the things you love.

- You'll see that you can think more clearly – and even see things in a different light!
- You'll see that when you walk, there is more spring to your step.

If you need to lose way more, don't worry. It will take longer but the habits you will develop in the first 30 days will carry you through the rest of your life.

# Chapter 1. Calorie Deficit: The End-all Be-all Of Weight Loss

So many of us have been there: we stop eating food we love, we cut down on what we eat to the point that we're miserable, and we even eat things we don't usually do, all for the pursuit of weight loss.

But the extra pounds just don't go away.

This book was created for precisely that – to guide you on how to effectively get rid of stubborn fat.

Yes, there is a way to get rid of those extra pounds – and it doesn't require hokey supplements or expensive surgery or backbreaking exercise.

This isn't to say that exercise isn't important. In fact, it's unarguable that physical activity is good for you. But you can still lose weight without working out (make no mistake: you *will* lose weight faster if you do).

This isn't to say that all supplements don't work. Some of them do and many of them facilitate weight loss by improving your workout performance.

But this book isn't about that – this book is about *diet*, which is the biggest factor in weight loss.

Now, let's talk about the Holy Grail of all diet regimens – **calorie deficit**.

### *What is calorie deficit?*

Calorie deficit occurs when energy intake (in the form of food) is less than your energy output.

You use up energy when you perform physical activity. In addition, the body uses up energy to perform basic functions so even when you're not doing anything like walking or jogging, you're still using up energy. This is called basal metabolism. Note that people who have considerable muscle mass have higher basal metabolic rate which means that even when they're at rest, they consume more energy.

### *The Weight Loss Formula*

The success of any diet regimen relies on whether or not there is calorie deficit. So even if you feel that you don't eat as much as you used to, or that you stopped eating certain kinds of food, you still wouldn't lose weight if the calorie count of what you're eating is higher than the calories you're burning.

This makes counting calories a habit worth developing if you want to lose weight.

Remember that the formula to losing weight is this:


Calorie intake < Calorie requirement per day

### *So how much of a deficit should you aim for?*

For the average woman, ideal daily calorie consumption is around 2000. This can change depending on your height and your physical activity. It's recommend that you use calorie calculators to determine your own weight loss targets.

To lose at least one pound a week, calorie intake should be reduced by about 500 calories per day (which means you should now be targeting a maximum of 1500 calories per day).

Healthy weight loss is around 1 to 2 pounds per week. It's possible to lose weight faster but many experts agree that 1 to 2 pounds per week is sustainable.

## *What can you eat with 1500 calories?*

Let's say your recommended daily calorie consumption for your weight loss target is now 1500 calories. You can already enjoy so much good food with that!

- You can have an avocado and arugula omelet for breakfast which is only about 340 calories. You can even enjoy some sugarless green tea with it, which is only 2 calories.

- You can then enjoy a 100-calorie snack, such as an apple or a cup of cheesy Brussels sprout chips.

- For lunch, you can have a yummy 300-calorie greek salad or a 340-calorie bacon-lettuce-tomato sandwich.

- For your afternoon snack, you can dip a cup of cucumber slices into some humus.
- For dinner, you can enjoy some seafood pasta which is only about 450 calories.

These examples are just to show you that you can eat well and still lose weight. It's all about the numbers. You will have to tweak your numbers depending on your height, weight, physical activity, and weight loss goals.

### *Counting calories*

Awareness of the calorie count of what you eat can help you stay on top of whether or not you're eating too much. Sadly, most people are not at all aware of the amount of calories that they consume.

Do you really have to count calories?

Yes you do, but there is no need to look up and memorize the precise calorie count of every food item there is.

We already have access to so much information. There is nutritional information found on the label foods. You can use apps to look them up. It only takes a few seconds to do so.

You can also look up the calorie count of thousands of food items. There are so many websites that provide the information. WebMd's food calorie counter is massive and is especially easy to use.

You just need to know the ballpark figures of the food items you would like to eat and those you usually eat and eventually, you can do the math in your head.

Download apps such as MyFitnessPal that can help you with counting calories. The calorie count of many food items are already part of the app's database.

Once you input a certain food type, its calorie count is automatically shown. This makes it easier to track if you still have enough room for certain meals. As long as you don't go over the recommended daily calorie requirement, you should be fine.

Using a calorie counter app works like a food diary. It helps you see the pattern in your diet.

Seeing which food contributes the most in your calorie intake will allow you to see the changes you need to make. You also get to see which foods have similar calorie counts. This makes it easier to look for substitutes in case you can't (or don't want to) consume that type of food today.

# Chapter 2. Winning The Mental Battle That Is Weight Loss

Now that we got the hard science of calorie counting out of the way, it's time for some real talk before we go into the kind of food you should be eating, and the yummy recipes you could try.

It's easy to say that you just need to keep track of calories. We can say all day that the key to weight loss is to just eat less and do more.

But there is a huge factor in that weight loss formula that isn't even really part of the equation:

*You* -- the human being behind the calories and the number of pounds to get rid of

All the talk about weight loss being all about a simple formula goes out the window when there's a human being involved – one with emotions, coping mechanisms, responsibilities, expectations, and all the little things that make up our lives.

The simple truth is that, if it's incredibly easy to lose weight, no one would be overweight.

But it's not easy to actually do it. And this is because weight loss is not just a physical battle. It has become a mental battle.

Every day, you have to face decisions on whether or not to eat just one more slice of pizza, one more sandwich, or one more helping of pasta.  And it takes mental fortitude to make the right decision.

Weight loss takes work. But the amazing thing is, anyone can do it. *You* can do it. You just need to win the mental battle to win the physical battle.

Weight loss is primarily about eating right to ensure calorie deficit, which in turn is about fundamental behaviors.

Losing weight is not just about eating the right food but also about how you position yourself toward the right behaviors.

Here's something you need to know: Will, like most things, can be strengthened. You need to reinforce your resolve through the right attitude and the right behaviors. That is what we will be talking about in this chapter.

Our focus will be to point out in how you could reprogram your mind through making small changes.

### Build the right habits

People struggle to lose weight because of certain habits. And some of those habits are not even related to the kind of food that we eat. This could sound surprising, but it is true.

There's a saying that goes "it takes 21 days to build a habit." Science says that is not true. A study published in the

European Journal of Social Psychology by a researcher from the University College London revealed that on average, it takes more than 2 months to build a habit.

So do your best to stick to the practices mentioned in this section for at least a few months. If you're going to start reducing the amount of snacks you eat, then try to do so continuously for at least 2 months. Do not worry about the time after that. Just focus first on how you can get it done for the first 2 months.

### *Practice Mindfulness*

Awareness of what you take in will help you realize just how much you've been eating – and how much you don't actually need. It also helps you assess whether or not you're eating food to cope with negative emotions such as stress and sadness, and not because you want to or need to.

This book is not about making you hate food and only eating some when you absolutely need to. In fact, that goes against what sustainable weight loss needs.

You can associate food with feeling good – but not in the sense that it automatically means your happiness and that eating more means drowning out the negative emotions.

You should enjoy food – but in the sense that the flavors make you feel grateful you're alive, or that it nourishes your body and mind and allows you to do so many things.

### *The size (of your plate) matters*

Sometimes, a change in perception is what you need. This is also helpful if you want to eat less. This can be achieved when you eat on a smaller plate.

People have the habit of always filling their plates with food, regardless of the size. Whether the plate is small or large, the person fills it up just the same.

Using a smaller plate gives the impression that you'll have a full serving. This influences the brain to tell the body that it had enough, and that it should stop eating. This significantly cuts the amount of calories that you intake to your body.

The color of the plate should also be considered. Research shows that bright-colored plates can make us eat less.

## *Eat at a slower pace*

Unless you are in a contest, eating should never be rushed.

Eating too fast may cause you to overeat. That's because the body does not easily realize that you're already full if you're eating too quickly. Your metabolism is unlikely to keep up with your food intake. Thus, your body thinks that you should still eat.

Chewing food slowly, on the other hand, helps in eating fewer calories. The body gets to process the food faster. If the body is able to tell if you're already full, you are less likely to overeat.

The production of hormones linked to weight loss is also improved when you eat slowly.

### Get enough sleep

Those who want to improve their overall health are advised to get 6 to 8 hours of sleep. This also works if you want to lose weight, and can even prevent weight gain.

Many researches have shown that around 55% of people who are deprived of enough sleep become obese. This number is higher if you are younger.

When you are deprived of sleep, your hormones related to your appetite are affected. This, in turn, leads to poor regulation of appetite. Also, when you don't get enough sleep, you feel tired.

Since you'll need energy to function, you're more likely to consume high-calorie foods. This kind of diet will cause you to become fat if you're not able to control it.

## *Small changes are better than no changes*

Do not be hard on yourself when you do lapse every once in a while. Remember that it's better to keep going. You lose a little momentum when your will breaks for a short while and you decide to eat more than usual, but that's nothing compared to what you will lose when you completely quit.

Be kind to yourself and just try again.

Losing weight is not an easy task. It requires dedication. However, it is not impossible. By adapting these new habits, you'll surely get on the right track when it comes to achieving this goal.

# The Ideal Weight Loss Diet

Now that we're through with the non-food and non-exercise tips, let's move on to things related to food.

As mentioned, weight loss can only happen if you have calorie deficit. This can only be achieved if you are closely monitoring your food intake.

Everything that will be listed here should be strictly followed and/or avoided. Only then can you start seeing results in your weight loss journey.

***What to eat/drink***

<u>Proteins</u>

Protein is the building block of muscles.

When you eat protein-rich food, your body is forced to digest and metabolize the fat stored in the other parts of your body.

A high-protein diet can also help suppress your appetite. That's because it makes you feel fuller.

You won't want to eat as much, so fewer calories are going into the body. Research even shows that those who have a high-protein diet consume 400 calories less than before.

With those facts presented, it's best that you start changing your diet. Include more protein-rich foods when you eat.

Even a hard-boiled egg or two for breakfast can work wonders to your metabolism and in burning calories.

Examples: Eggs, meat, fish, poultry


<u>Whole foods</u>

Whole foods are foods that have undergone as little processing as possible. They are naturally filling.

Whole foods are also known for the essential nutrients that they contain allowing your body to function well. They also do not contain a lot of additives such as extra sugars which can cause weight gain.

Raw fruits and vegetables are the most common examples of whole foods. They contain fiber and lots of nutrients, helping your body to function properly.

Fruits and veggies have low energy density. This only means that even if you have large servings, you're not taking in a lot of calories. Just don't eat too much and you'll be fine.

Examples: Unprocessed fruits, nuts, vegetables, whole grains, eggs


Fiber

Fiber slows the rate at which the body absorbs sugar. As a result, you prevent your blood sugar levels from rising too quickly. This means that you can manage your appetite better. As a bonus, fiber helps reduce cholesterol levels and promote regular bowel movement.

Examples: Whole grains, brown rice, berries, bran cereal, beans


## Cruciferous Vegetables

Cruciferous vegetables are low-calorie but satisfying, thanks to their fiber content. They also contain lots of protein and can complement lots of dishes.

Examples: broccoli, Brussels sprouts, cauliflower, kale, cabbage


## Seafood

Seafood contains good amounts of iodine which is crucial for the proper functioning of your thyroid gland. The thyroid regulates your metabolism so having enough iodine means that your metabolism will keep running at its optimal levels.

Fatty fish such as mackerel, salmon and trout is especially recommended because it contains lots of omega-3 fatty acids which are good for your heart.

Examples: mackerel, salmon, shrimp, sardines, herring, trout

<u>Unsweetened coffee or tea</u>

Many people drink coffee to wake up. However, coffee is more than that. This drink not only has caffeine; it also has antioxidants and other compounds beneficial to the body.

Drinking caffeinated coffee can boost your metabolism as high as 11%. It's also this same component that reduces the risk of getting type 2 diabetes for as high as 50%!

The catch, though, is that you have to drink unsweetened coffee, or at least use very little sugar.

Unsweetened green tea is also an option. Green tea has been linked to selective fat burning, targeting belly fat. Research shows that up to 17% harmful belly fat can be burned with the help of unsweetened green tea.

It's also known to increase the body's usage of energy by up to 4%. Yes, using energy up can cause you to be hungry faster. But this also means that your body doesn't stock up too much calories. Thus, the development of fat is prevented.


## Water

Aside from unsweetened coffee and green tea, the only thing that you can drink without getting extra calories is water. This is just one of the things why it can help with weight loss.

It's also surprising that when you drink 17 ounces of water, the burning of calories in your body may increase by up to 30% for the next hour.

Calorie intake can be reduced because of water because it makes you feel fuller.

Coconut Oil

Use coconut oil as a substitute for bad fats such as trans fats.

You should not completely cut out fat from your diet. After all, fat is good for you and is a better source of energy compared to carbs if your goal is weight loss.

There are healthier alternatives to some fats used for cooking, and one of those is coconut oil.

Coconut oil contains medium-chain triglycerides. The body metabolizes MCTs in a different way. Research also shows that coconut oil can slightly boost your metabolism. Thus, you get to burn calories a little bit faster. It can also influence your body to eat less, and therefore consume fewer calories. Surprisingly, it can also reduce harmful belly fat.

Modify your diet so that you can use coconut oil instead of fats like butter.


### *What to Avoid*

<u>Any processed food</u>

This kind of food is known for having a lot of additives such as sugar, fats, salt, or even calories. And to experience the benefits of eating whole foods, this should be out of your diet.

Our brain likes sweet and salty foods. That's why "comfort foods" are either sweet or a bit salty. And most processed foods taste either one or the other, making it difficult to stop eating. To avoid eating so much processed food, make sure there are healthy foods that can be readily eaten in your kitchen.

<u>Sugar</u>

The two main forms of carbohydrates are sugars and starches. In fact, all sugars are technically carbohydrates. However, there is bad sugar and good sugar. Bad sugars refer to those that make up simple carbs and good sugars refer to those that make up complex carbs.

Sugar is generally linked to the development of many diseases such as type 2 diabetes, heart disease, and even cancer.

With so many processed food sold nowadays, it's highly possible that you're consuming sugar without knowing it. Ready-made spaghetti sauce and breakfast cereals, for example, contain lots of sugars.

In fact, it's shown that the average person is consuming an additional 15 teaspoons of sugar in a day just from the usual food they eat!

Examples: agave nectar, high-fructose corn syrup, sucrose, glucose, corn syrup, raw sugar

<u>Liquid calories</u>

Another thing that you should get rid of on your road to weight loss are sugary beverages. Some examples include soft drinks, chocolate milk, energy drinks, and fruit juices.

While it is technically liquid, it contains a lot of sugar, which increases the risk of obesity. This is especially true for children. In fact, one study reveals that children are 60% more likely to become obese for each day that they consume liquid calories.

Examples: Soda, sugary/commercially-produced fruit drinks

<u>Refined carbs</u>

Yes, we need carbs so that we can have energy. But when it comes to refined carbs, your consumption should be limited.

The reason for that is because refined carbs had their fiber and most of their beneficial nutrients removed. When foods undergo the refining process, only the easily digestible carbohydrates remain. While this is great for adding a sudden burst of energy to your body, it increases your tendency to overeat.

Examples: white rice, white flour, white bread, sweets and snacks, pastries, breakfast cereals, and even pasta.

Weight loss heavily depends on the food that you eat. See how you can change your diet to include as many healthy foods as possible. The same goes for cutting out foods that don't help with your goal.

Losing weight and dieting is a commitment. It should be done consistently if you want to get results, just like how other things in life are.

# Try Intermittent Fasting

One effective dieting plan that gained hype over the past years is intermittent fasting.

With intermittent fasting, the person deliberately chooses not to eat for a period of time. Not too different from the usual fasting that many people already know.

However, with this method, the person is not forced to fast for the whole day. Rather, there is only a period of time during that day when you will be allowed to eat. After that period has passed, eating is again restricted.

People fast every day. That's how the term breakfast was coined. That meal literally breaks the fast that you had while you were sleeping. You already fast every day, and if you want to lose weight, you will benefit from fasting for a longer period of time for better effects.

### *How does the body work when fasting?*

To better understand how the body works when fasting and how it contributes to weight loss, let's delve into its science first.

The typical way on how our body works in relation to food is this:

- When we feel hungry, we eat food

- Once we've eaten, our body breaks down the carbohydrates in food and turns it into insulin.

- Once the insulin level in our bloodstream is increased, our body uses whatever it can depending on our activity. The rest are stored as either sugar in our liver or is converted as fat. The sugar stored in our liver is limited, but can easily be used by the body. On the other hand, sugar that is converted to fat isn't easily used by the body, but there is no limit to how much can be stored.

The points above describe what happens when we are in a state of high insulin, or after we just ate something. It also described how we accumulate fat.

Fasting, on the other hand, works the other way around. That's because when we fast, the body first uses up the insulin that is found in our bloodstream. Once that insulin has been used up, the body starts to access the excess sugar found in your liver. When you take it up a notch and still not consume food, that's the time when the body uses up the sugar that was converted into fat. This explains why weight loss becomes possible with fasting.

When you fast continuously (day after day), the body becomes more trained to burn your fats into energy that it can use once it runs out of insulin in the bloodstream and the liver. Think of this process as the way of your body to use all of its resources so that it will continue to function properly.

Fasting also teaches the body to become more sensitive to insulin. When the body is sensitive to insulin, it uses the energy from the food you eat more efficiently. It automatically directs that energy to important areas of your system so that you will stay functional even if deprived of food.

## Variations of intermittent fasting

Because many have supported the idea of this diet plan, numerous variations of intermittent fasting has been introduced.

These variations mostly refer to the number of hours or days when you should be fasting.

The most common fasting variations are as follows:

- 16:8 fasting - for this plan, you are required to fast for 16 hours a day, followed by an 8 hour window period wherein you can consume food. The 8 hours of sleep is counted as a fasting period.

- 20:4 fasting - same as above; this time, though, you have to fast for 20 hours and only allot 4 hours for eating.

- 5:2 diet - in this method, the person is allowed to eat a regular 2000 calorie diet for 5 days. However, for their fasting days, the person's calorie intake will be limited so that weight loss could happen.

You can also just stick to the natural fasting period that happens when you sleep. You can also still eat breakfast, but delay it just for a few hours. This way, you get to extend your fasting a little bit and limit your window for eating hours. It's even possible for you to not skip meals and still experience weight loss! For example, an 8 AM to 6 PM eating window will allow you to consume all meals but still have a significant number of hours for fasting.

With intermittent fasting, the key is to limit the number of hours that you can eat. That way, you can significantly restrict the amount of calories coming into your body.

Before adapting this diet plan, it's best to consult to a doctor. If you have a condition that would cause harm if you miss a meal, then this diet plan is not for you.

In case any of the routines mentioned above is too extreme for you, no worries. The meal plan we prepared in the next chapter will not force you to go on this fasting regimen. We will merely make recommendations on when you can start fasting after the first week but you can still enjoy your usual 3 meals.

# Sample Meal Plans For Weight Loss

If you're just starting your weight loss journey, you'll need all the help you can get, so we developed a meal plan that would help you integrate healthy, low calorie recipes into your diet.

Note that a few of these recipes make more than 1 serving so please adjust amount of ingredients according to the number of people you're preparing for. You can also put some of the food in the fridge and microwave it at a later time.

Although we've mentioned that intermittent fasting is a good way to lose weight, we do not recommend it for the first week. Your body is still adjusting to the reduced calories that you're taking in.

Thus, even without fasting, there's a huge possibility that some pounds will be shed off of your initial weight.

We encourage you to try the meal plan we have prepared. For the next 30 days, you'll get to enjoy making the recipes here. Your first week should be awesome so we chose yummy recipes that do not have more than 500 calories.

Because many of these recipes are low-calorie, you can even enjoy 100-calorie snacks in between meals. We've provided some recipes at the end of the recipes section.

## *Week 1 Meal Plan*

These recipes for the following meals can be found in the next pages.

|  | Breakfast | Lunch | Dinner |
| --- | --- | --- | --- |
| Monday | Coconut cookies | Chicken spring rolls in a jar | Honey Garlic Shrimp |
| Tuesday | Green smoothie | Burgers made from grass-fed beef | Stir fried chicken and broccoli |
| Wednes day | Matcha green tea bites | Beef wraps spiced with cumin | Salmon and veggies |
| Thursda | Keto | Keto-style | Zucchini |

| y | cheese roll-ups | Asian beef salad | noodles |
|---|---|---|---|
| Friday | Coconut porridge | Keto-friendly quesadillas | Keto pizza |
| Saturday | Mushroom omelettes | Artichokes and shrimp plate | Seared Chicken and Quinoa Salad |
| Sunday | Breakfast burrito | Healthy chef's salad | Home-style chicken noodle soup |

<u>**Breakfast Recipes**</u>

*Coconut cookies*

With this recipe, you're able to get your supply of protein first thing in the morning with the help of the protein powder. The shredded coconuts will be your source of fiber.

Servings: 12

Calories: 130 per cookie.

Ingredients:

- 2 tablespoons of coconut oil

- 1 ½ cups of shredded coconut flakes

- 1 teaspoon of cinnamon

- 1 teaspoon vanilla

- ½ cup of sunflower seeds

- ½ cup of high quality protein powder

- ¼ cup of honey

- ⅛ cup of water

Instructions:

1. Start by preheating the oven to 300 degrees.

2. Next, place the coconut flakes in a large bowl, then add all the ingredients.

3. Using a wooden spoon, mix the ingredients together.

4. Once everything is thoroughly mixed, take small handfuls of the mixture and roll it into a little ball. Place it on a baking sheet lined in parchment and flatten it out.

5. Place in the oven and bake for 15 minutes.

*Green smoothie*

Many people start their day with a smoothie, but some of them start with the wrong smoothie. Here's a healthier green smoothie version.

Smoothies won't upset your stomach after fasting. It also preps you for a solid meal.

Avocado has lots of vitamins and minerals and is yummy to boot. It contains a lot of calorie (1 medium sized avocado has over 300 calories), but you can use just half and set the other half for the next day. It also has enough fiber to make you feel full until your next meal.

Servings: 1

Calories: 280.

Ingredients:

- 1/2 avocado
- 1 cup of coconut milk
- 1 cup of spinach or kale
- 1 tablespoon of chia seeds
- A handful of berries

Instructions

Just mix all of these in the blender and pour yourself a smoothie once everything is mixed thoroughly.

*Matcha bites*

This quick recipe is perfect if you don't have a lot of time to prepare food. Now you have a recipe that you can grab and easily consume while you're on your way to work. This would make for a great snack as well.

You can add matcha into food and enjoy the same benefits you'd have gotten from tea.

The amount of maple syrup entirely depends on your preferences. It's recommended that you use less of it.

Servings: 8-10

Calorie count per serving 120-150

Ingredients:

- 1 tablespoon of matcha green tea
- 1 tablespoon of coconut oil
- 1 cup of shredded coconut, unsweetened
- 2 tablespoons of maple syrup
- 4 tablespoons of almond flour

Instructions:

1. Place all your ingredients in the food processor and blend.
2. Once everything is thoroughly mixed, roll the mixture into at least 1-inch diameter balls.
3. Optional: Sprinkle coconut flakes into the matcha balls.
4. Store what you're unable to eat in the refrigerator.

*Keto cheese roll-ups*

This recipe only involves a few ingredients, and is easy to prepare.

Calorie count: 334 for all rollups

Ingredients

- 8 ounces of sliced provolone or cheddar cheese
- 2 ounces of butter

Instructions:

1. Lay out the cheese slices on your cutting board.

2.  Slice butter using a cheese slicer,
    or use your kitchen knife and
    slice really thin pieces of butter.
3.  Cover the cheese slices with
    butter, then roll it up. Enjoy!


Optional: Feel free to add salt flakes, paprika powder, or even finely chopped herbs (such as parsley).

*Coconut porridge*

Porridge is the kind of food that's usually made with rice. But did you know that you can take out the rice and use coconut instead?

Servings: 1

Calorie count: 491

Ingredients:

- 1 ounce of coconut oil (butter can be used as an alternative)
- 1 tablespoon of coconut flour
- 4 tablespoons of coconut cream
- 1 egg
- A pinch of salt
- A pinch of psyllium husk powder

Instructions:

- Start by adding all the ingredients on a non-stick pan. Mix everything well and cook over low heat.
- Stir the mixture constantly until the desired texture is achieved.
- Serve the porridge using coconut cream or milk. Feel free to eat your porridge with berries, fresh or frozen.

If you have excess coconut milk, save it for your next smoothie. Coconut milk can make your smoothie thicker, richer, and more filling.

*Mushroom omelettes*

The omelette is also a common breakfast recipe in most homes. But if you want this simple recipe to be healthier, why not make mushroom omelettes instead?

Servings: 1

Calorie count: 461 (For some people, even half of the output for this recipe is enough)

Ingredients:

- 3 eggs
- 3 mushrooms (any kind
- 1 ounce of shredded cheese
- 1 ounce of butter (will be used for frying)
- 1/5 of a whole yellow onion

Instructions

1. Put eggs in a mixing bowl. Add salt and pepper. Using a fork, whisk the eggs until it becomes frothy and smooth. Feel free to add salt and other spices to get your desired taste.
2. Melt the butter in your frying pan. Put the egg mixture once the butter melts.
3. Once the egg starts to cook and get firm, but there's still some raw egg on top, sprinkle the cheese, onion, and mushroom.
4. With a spatula, ease the edges of the omelet. Fold the omelet over in half. Once the underside becomes golden brown in color, turn off the heat, remove the pan,

then slide out the omelet going to
your plate.

*Breakfast burrito*

This breakfast burrito can give you the energy you need for the entire morning.

Servings: 1

Calories: 290

Ingredients

- 8" whole wheat tortilla
- 3 pieces scrambled egg whites
- 1 tablespoon of chopped sweet onion
- 1 tablespoon of salsa
- 1/2 cup of diced tomatoes
- 1/4 cup of yellow bell pepper, diced
- 1/4 cup of unsalted canned black beans

## Instructions

Just place all ingredients inside the tortilla and wrap accordingly.

# Lunch Recipes

Not everyone who follows intermittent fasting consumes breakfast, but all of them definitely have lunch. Here, we'll give you some lunch ideas to get started with your diet.

*Chicken spring rolls in a jar*

A lot of meals are being placed in jars nowadays so that they are handier. Many of these meals in a jar, however, are cakes and preserved food. Why not break that trend and use the jar for healthier foods? This recipe in particular is healthy and easy to make.

Calorie count: 450 calories, with 27 grams of protein

Each jar lasts up to 5 days if kept in the fridge.

Ingredients:

- 2 cups of cooked vermicelli noodles
- 1 pound of ground turkey or chicken
- soy sauce (separated into 2 tablespoons and 2 teaspoons)
- 2 cloves of garlic, minced
- 1 tablespoon of ginger, minced
- 1 tablespoon of sesame oil
- 1 cup of cucumber, sliced into "matchstick" sizes
- 1 cup of sliced red pepper
- A bag of coleslaw
- ½ cup of sweet chili sauce

- ⅓ cup of chopped cilantro (you can also use or add basil and fresh mint)
- ¼ cup sesame seeds
- Sriracha to taste

Instructions:

1. In a large skillet, heat the sesame oil over medium to high heat.
2. Add the ground chicken/turkey and 2 tablespoons of soy sauce, then cook for around 2 to 3 minutes.
3. Add the ginger and garlic, then continue to sauté for 7 minutes, or until chicken is cooked.
4. Remove the chicken once it's cooked. Add the coleslaw and 2 teaspoons of soy sauce with the

other ingredients in the pan. Continue to sauté for 2 to 3 minutes, or until coleslaw is slightly wilted.

5.  Cook the vermicelli noodles based on the directions specified in the package. It's usually cooked in boiling water for around 2 to 3 minutes.

6.  In your mason jars, start pouring a little of the chili sauce. The cooked chicken should be divided among your jars. Place the coleslaw, cucumber, and red pepper next. The vermicelli noodles, sesame seeds, and fresh herbs should be placed on top. You can also add sriracha and soy sauce if you want to.

7. Chicken and turkey are good substitutes for pork because they don't contain a lot of fat. You also get the benefits of the vegetables mixed in your food. Vermicelli, though a kind of noodle, contains fewer carbohydrates.

*Burger patties made from grass-fed beef*

Do you feel like eating a burger but you're thinking twice about doing so because it might hinder your weight loss goal?

Here's a recipe for a guilt-free burger.

And since these are burgers, you can involve other members of the family with your regimen. You can even encourage them to eat healthily!

Servings: 4 patties

Calorie count: 220 per patty

Calorie count with hamburger buns and condiments: 350

Calorie count With Cheese: 460

Ingredients

- ½ pound grass-fed beef; ground
- ½ pound of ground grass-fed beef liver
- ½ teaspoon of cumin powder
- ½ teaspoon of garlic powder
- Salt and pepper to taste

Instructions

1. Start by mixing together all the ingredients in a bowl. Once the ingredients are thoroughly mixed, form them into patties based on your desired size.
2. In a skillet, heat the cooking oil on medium-high heat. Once hot, cook the patties until it reaches your desired doneness. You can

store the cooked patties in the fridge for up to four days.

3. Beef is a rich source of protein. If you eat it along with leafy greens, your meal will be packed with nutrients. You can make your own dressing and use it in the burger so that it will meet your desired taste.

*Beef wraps spiced with cumin*

Here's another beef recipe that will surely help you lose weight. And it's not just because of the protein. It's also about cumin.

Cumin is known to help people who are having problems with indigestion. It also contains other beneficial components such as iron and antioxidants.

Calorie count: 375 (4 grams of carbohydrates, 30 grams of protein)

This recipe is easy to make and bring to work.

Ingredients:

- 8 pieces of large cabbage leaves (either Napa or savoy cabbage)

- ⅔ pounds of ground beef
- 2 teaspoons cumin
- 1 to 2 tablespoons of coconut oil
- 4 cloves of garlic, minced
- 2 tablespoons of chopped cilantro
- ¼ of an onion, chopped into small dice
- 1 red bell pepper, diced into small pieces
- 1 teaspoon of minced ginger
- Salt and pepper

Instructions:

1. Use the coconut oil to sauté onions, peppers, and ground beef on medium heat.
2. Once the beef is cooked, add the remaining ingredients except for the cabbage.

3. Fill a large pot with water until it is ¾ full. Bring that to a boil.

4. Blanch the cabbage leaves, submerging them into the boiling water for at least 20 seconds using tongs. After being soaked in boiling water, immediately plunge them in cold water. Drain the liquid and place it on a plate.

5. Add the beef mixture onto the lettuce leaf, then fold it until it looks like a roll.

*Keto-style Asian beef salad*

This salad combines the benefits of both veggies and beef. At the same time, you're not taking in carbs, which helps in your weight loss goal and getting back those curves.

Though there are a lot of ingredients, it's relatively easy to make. In addition, you can be sure that you are consuming a complete meal.

Note that this recipe is for multiple servings so it's ideal for those who are preparing meals for multiple people. You can adjust the ingredients or set some servings aside for dinner or the following day's breakfast.

Servings: 3

Calorie Count: 378

Ingredients

For the beef:

- ⅔ pounds of ribeye steak
- A teaspoon of chili flakes
- A tablespoon of fish sauce
- A tablespoon of olive oil
- 1 tablespoon of grated ginger

For the salad:

- 3 ounces of lettuce
- 3 ounces of cherry tomatoes
- 2 ounces of cucumber
- 2 pieces of scallions
- 1 tablespoon of sesame seeds

- ½ piece of red onions
- Fresh cilantro

For the sesame mayonnaise

- 1 egg yolk; must be at room temperature
- 1 tablespoon of sesame oil
- A teaspoon of Dijon mustard
- Half tablespoon of lime juice
- ½ cup of of light olive oil or avocado oil

Instructions:

1. Start making the sesame mayonnaise. You can do this by mixing the mustard and egg yolk in a bowl.

2. Slowly add the avocado or olive oil while you whisk the mixture continuously, either by using a hand mixer, by hand, or with an immersion blender. Add the lime juice, spices, and sesame oil when the mayonnaise emulsified. Set aside the mayonnaise first.

3. Start preparing the beef. You can do this by mixing all the other ingredients to make the marinade and pouring that into a plastic bag. After making the marinade, mix the beef in and marinate it for at least 15 minutes. Let it sit at room temperature.

4. To make the salad, chop all vegetables into bite-sized pieces (except for the scallions). Divide

the chopped vegetables into two plates.

5. Heat a medium frying pan. Once heated, toast the sesame seeds for a few minutes. Set it aside when it becomes fragrant and lightly browned.

6. Use paper towels to pat the beef dry. Make sure that both sides are dried out. Fry each side for a minute or two on high heat. Cook the meat until it's medium (more prefered) or well-done.

7. When you're done frying the beef, use that same pan for frying the scallions for at least a minute.

8. Start slicing the meat thinly. Place that and the scallions on top of your vegetables. Serve the salad with the sesame

mayonnaise and the roasted sesame seeds.

*Keto-friendly quesadillas*

This quesadilla recipe comes with a twist.

You'll be using coconut flour, you can be sure that you're not raking up calories and carbs. It's also a good source of protein, healthy fats, and fiber.

And since you'll also be making your own tortillas, you can be sure that it will be free from carbs!

Makes 8 slices

Calories per slice: 125

Ingredients:

For the tortilla

- 2 egg whites
- 2 eggs
- A tablespoon of coconut flour
- 6 ounces of cream cheese
- 1.5 teaspoons of psyllium husk powder
- ½ teaspoon of salt

For the filling

- A tablespoon of olive oil (to be used for frying)
- An ounce of leafy greens
- 5 ounces of grated Mexican cheese

Instructions:

For the tortilla:

1. Get the oven preheated to 400 degrees Fahrenheit.

2. Beat the egg whites and the eggs together until those become fluffy. Throw in the cream cheese and continue beating the mixture until it becomes smooth.

3. In a small bowl, combine the coconut flour, salt, and psyllium husk powder and mix it well. Add this into the egg mixture while continuously beating it.

4. Allow the batter to sit for a few minutes so that you can check its thickness (which should be like a pancake batter). Add more psyllium husk powder if the batter isn't thick enough.

5. Place parchment paper on your baking sheet. Using a spatula, spread the batter on the parchment paper and shape them

to look like big squares. In case you want round tortillas, you can fry those instead like pancakes.

6. Place the baking sheet on the upper rack and bake it between 5 and 7 minutes. It's done cooking when the edges become a little brown. Make sure not to overcook, as you will end up with a tortilla that has a burned bottom.

7. Cut the tortilla into smaller pieces.

For the quesadilla:

1. Start heating a small but non-stick skillet. Add butter or oil if you want to. Then, put the tortilla in the pan.

2. Sprinkle the tortilla with cheese, followed by leafy greens, followed by more cheese, and topped by another tortilla.

3. Fry the quesadillas for at least a minute for both sides. When the cheese melts, the quesadillas are cooked.

*Artichokes and shrimp plate*

Here's a quick and easy lunch that makes use of shrimps.

Aside from containing dietary fibers, it's also a good source of vitamin C, K, and folate. It also contains a lot of antioxidants.

It even ranks 7th out of the 20 food types listed by the USDA when it comes to the antioxidants that it has. Keep your free radical levels in check while you stay healthy and within your target weight.

Servings 4

Calories: 387

Ingredients:

- 14 ounces of canned artichokes
- 10 ounces of shrimp (cooked and peeled)
- 6 pieces of sun-riped tomatoes
- 4 tablespoons of olive oil
- 4 eggs
- 1.5 ounce of baby spinach
- ½ cup of mayonnaise

Instructions:

1. Start by cooking the eggs. Lower each egg carefully into boiling water for at least 4 to 8 minutes. Depending on your preferred egg (soft or hard boiled), it should be submerged in water for a specific amount of time.

2. Once you're done cooking the eggs, submerge it in cold water for a minute or two. This makes it easier for you to remove the egg shells.

3. Place the shrimp, eggs, mayonnaise, artichokes, tomatoes, and spinach on your plate.

4. Use the olive oil by drizzling it on top of the spinach.

*Healthy chef's salad*

Salad is still a forerunner when it comes to healthy recipes. To make your own 400-calorie salad, you need to prepare this salad.

Servings:1

Calories: 375

Ingredients:

- 2 cups of romaine lettuce
- 2 ounces of sliced turkey breast
- 5 pieces of grape tomatoes
- 1 hard-boiled egg
- 2 slices of red onion
- 1/3 cup of sliced avocado

- 2 teaspoons of red wine vinegar
- 1 tablespoon of olive oil

Instructions:

Simply mix all ingredients in a bowl.

Optional: Serve with 2 tangerines.

<u>**Dinner recipes**</u>

Your day is about to end, but it doesn't mean that you can whatever you want because you're fasting anyways.

These dinner recipes will surely satisfy your cravings for good food but still help you lose weight.

*Honey Garlic Shrimp*

Seafood, the main ingredient of this recipe, is a great source of protein and iodine.

Servings: 4

Calories: 265

Ingredients:

- a pound of uncooked shrimp. It must also be peeled and deveined (removing the "vein" that runs along the back of the shrimp)
- 1 tablespoon of garlic, minced
- 2 teaspoons of olive oil
- ⅓ cup honey
- ¼ cup soy sauce
- 1 teaspoon fresh ginger, minced (optional)
- Chopped green onion (for garnish, also optional)

Instructions:

1. Start by whisking the garlic, ginger, honey, and soy sauce in a medium-sized bowl. This will serve as your marinade.

2. Next, place the shrimp in a large tupperware or a zipped-top bag. Use half of the marinade and pour it on top of the shrimp. Stir the mixture or shake the container, then marinate it for at least 15 minutes in the fridge. It can be marinated for up to 12 hours. Cover the remaining marinade mixture and put it in the fridge.

3. Once the shrimp has been marinated, place the olive oil in the skillet and set the temperature of the stove to medium high. Once oil is heated, place the shrimp and discard the used marinade. Cook one side of the shrimp first until it turns pink (around 45 seconds) then flip it

over. Pour the remaining marinade and cook for at least 1 minute.

4. Serve the shrimp and the cooked marinade. Use the green onions for garnishing.

*Stir fried chicken and broccoli*

You can prepare and cook the dish in as little as 30 minutes! It also makes use of Broccoli which is rich in fiber a good source of Vitamin K and C, potassium, and folate.

Servings: 4

Calories: 308 calories per serving

Ingredients

- 2 cups of small broccoli florets
- A pound of boneless and skinless chicken breast. Cut it into approximately 1 inch pieces
- A cup of sliced mushrooms. This can be replaced by more broccoli if you don't like mushrooms

- Vegetable oil (must be separated in 1 tablespoon and 1 teaspoon)
- ¼ cup of chicken broth or water
- ¼ cup oyster sauce
- 1 teaspoon cornstarch
- 1 teaspoon soy sauce
- 1 teaspoon sugar
- 1 teaspoon of minced garlic
- 2 teaspoons of minced ginger
- 2 teaspoons of toasted sesame oil
- Salt and pepper

Instructions:

1. In a large frying pan, heat 1 teaspoon of vegetable oil over medium heat. Put the mushrooms and broccoli and cook it for about 4 minutes, or

until the vegetables become tender.

2. Add the garlic and ginger. Cook for another 30 seconds. Remove the vegetables from the pan and transfer it on a plate. Cover.

3. Using a paper towel, wipe the oil off the pan. Once oil is wiped off, pour 1 tablespoon of cooking oil and turn the temperature of the stove to high.

4. Using the salt and pepper, season the chicken pieces. Lay each piece to the pan in a single layer. In case all pieces don't fit in the pan, separate the cooking into batches. Cook the chicken for around 3 to 4 minutes for each side, making sure that it's golden brown and is thoroughly cooked.

5. Add the vegetables that you initially set aside to the pan. Cook for around 2 minutes or until the vegetables are warm again.

6. In a bowl, mix together the chicken broth, oyster sauce, sesame oil, sugar, and soy sauce. In a smaller bowl, mix the cornstarch to one tablespoon of cold water.

7. Pour the mixture with the oyster sauce on the vegetables and chicken, then cook for another 30 seconds.

8. Add the cornstarch mixture and bring it to a bowl. Cook it for about 1 minute or until the sauce starts to thicken.

*Salmon and veggies*

Salmon gets a lot of attention because it packs a lot of vitamins and minerals. It's also known for its great taste.

Here is a salmon recipe that you can easily whip up.

Servings: 4

Calories per serving: 300

Ingredients:

- A pound of salmon (can also be used on other fish of your choice)
- 2 tablespoons of ghee (ingredient similar to clarified butter and is made by heating up butter made from grass-fed cattle)

- 2 tablespoons of fresh lemon juice
- 4 cloves of finely diced garlic

Instructions:

1. Preheat your oven to 400 degrees Fahrenheit
2. Mix the garlic, ghee, and lemon juice together
3. Place the salmon in a foil and pour the ghee and lemon juice mixture over it. Once poured, wrap the fish with the foil. Place it on a baking sheet afterwards.
4. Bake the salmon for at least 15 minutes, or until it's cooked through.
5. As for the vegetable, that depends on what you like with your

salmon. Any cruciferous vegetable such as broccoli would be great. Place it in the oven as well.

*Zucchini noodles*

If you want to whip up a slightly different pasta dish for a party, try this recipe. This recipe is good for 10 people so you might want to adjust the recipe if you're cooking for fewer people.

Servings: 10

Calories per serving: 290

Ingredients:

- 30 ounces zucchini
- 10 ounces of diced pancetta or bacon
- 3 ounces of parmesan cheese, grated
- 4 egg yolks
- 1 tablespoon of butter

- 1 and ¼ cup of heavy whipping cream
- ¼ cup of mayonnaise
- Salt and pepper to taste
- Chopped fresh parsley

Instructions:

1. In a saucepan, pour heavy cream and bring that into a boil. Lower heat and boil it again for a few minutes.
2. In a separate pan, fry the bacon in butter until it becomes crispy. Set aside bacon fat.
3. Mix the mayonnaise and heavy cream. Add salt and pepper until you get your desired taste.
4. Make zucchini spirals using a spiralizer. In case you don't have

one, you can also use a potato peeler and make zucchini strips.

5. Add the zucchini noodles with the cream sauce. Divide the batch that you made into four plates. Top the zucchini noodles with egg yolks parsley, bacon, and top it with newly grated parmesan.

6. Use the bacon fat that you've initially set aside and drizzle it over the zucchini noodles.

*Keto pizza*

You've probably ordered pizza for dinner. Unfortunately, it contains a lot of carbs. Fortunately, there a way to eat pizza and still be able to reach your weight loss goal.

Whether or not you're on a keto diet, this recipe is worth trying out. Note that this one has a little over 500 calories though.

Servings: 8

Calories: 570

Ingredients:

For the crust:

- 6 ounces of mozzarella or provolone, preferably shredded
- 4 eggs

For the toppings:

1. 1 and ½ pounds of pepperoni
2. Olives
3. A teaspoon of dried oregano
4. 3 tablespoons of tomato paste
5. 5 ounces of shredded cheese

Instructions:

1. Get your oven preheated to 400 degrees Fahrenheit
2. Make the crust first. This is done by first cracking the eggs into a medium bowl. Add the shredded

cheese, and combine it thoroughly while still mixing.

3. Use the spatula so that this batter can be spread accordingly into the baking sheet.

4. Bake the pizza for around 15 minutes, or until the crust becomes golden brown. Remove it from the oven and let it cool for at least 1 to 2 minutes.

5. Once done with the crust, preheat the oven again.

6. Spread the tomato paste on the crust. For the oregano, it can be used as a sprinkle on top. After the oregano, put more cheese, pepperoni, and olives.

7. Bake the pizza for at least 5 to 10 minutes, or until it becomes golden.

*Seared Chicken and Quinoa Salad*

For those who want a protein boost, the combination of chicken and quinoa will do the trick.

Quinoa has quite a reputation as being a highly nutritious food - and for good reason. It has high fiber content, low glycemic index, and gluten-free. Keep in mind, though, that quinoa is still high in carbs, so its consumption should still be moderated.

Servings:  4

Calories per serving: 379

Ingredients:

For the Chicken:

- 2 skinless and boneless chicken breasts, cut into bite-sized pieces
- A tablespoon of extra virgin olive oil
- 1/2 teaspoon salt
- 1/4 teaspoon of black pepper

For the salad:

- 2/3 cup of rinsed quinoa
- 4 cups of baby arugula
- 1 cucumber, diced
- 1 red bell pepper, chopped and seeds must be removed
- 1/2 teaspoon salt
- 1/4 cup of diced celery


For the dressing, here's what you need:

- 1 clove of minced garlic
- 1/4 teaspoon of sea salt

- 1/4 teaspoon of black pepper
- 1 teaspoon of Dijon mustard
- 2 teaspoons of honey
- 1 tablespoon of balsamic vinegar
- 2 tablespoons of extra-virgin olive oil

Instructions:

For the chicken:

In a heavy bottomed skillet, heat the oil over medium high heat. Put the chicken in and cook it until meat is browned. Season it with salt and pepper. Once chicken is cooked thoroughly, set aside.

For the quinoa:

In a medium saucepan, put the quinoa and salt along with 1 1/3 cup of water.

Bring it to a boil, then cover the saucepan and reduce the heat. Continue to simmer until all liquid is absorbed.

Let it stay covered for 5 minutes before removing the lid. Put the other vegetables in a large bowl, then add the quinoa. Mix well.

To make the salad:

Place all ingredients in a jar with a lid. Shake the lid until everything is mixed well. Add it to the salad along with the chicken. Serve the salad warm or cold.

*Home-style chicken noodle soup*

For the last recipe of this week, you can keep it simple and make this healthier version of the chicken noodle soup.

Servings: 4

Calories: 330

Ingredients:

- 3 large pieces of skinless and boneless chicken breasts
- 4 cups of chicken stock or broth, preferably natural-made
- 2 cups of whole grain noodles
- 2 cups of water
- A cup of canned coconut milk
- 2 pieces of chopped celery stalks
- 2 pieces of chopped carrots

- 1 piece of minced garlic clove
- 2 cups of frozen peas
- A cup of frozen corn
- 2 tablespoons of minced onions
- 3 teaspoons of Kosher salt
- 2 teaspoons of black pepper
- 1/2 teaspoon of dried thyme

Instructions:

1. Place all ingredients except for the noodles in the slow cooker. Cook it for 4 hours on high and 6 hours for low.
2. After that's done, remove the chicken, shred it, then put it back in the slow cooker, this time, with the cooked noodles. Heat it for 5 more minutes, and then serve it.

# **Bonus recipes: Delightful 100-Calorie Snacks**

*Mini Chocolate-Strawberry Yogurt Bars*

Servings: 32

Ingredients:

- 1 and ½ cups strawberries, sliced
- 3 cups Greek yogurt
- ¼ cup honey or maple syrup
- ¼ cup mini chocolate chips
- 1 tsp. vanilla extract

Instructions:

1. Mix yogurt, vanilla, and honey (or maple syrup) in a bowl. Stir well.
2. Line a rimmed baking sheet or a baking pan with parchment paper
3. Transfer yogurt mixture into baking sheet and form a 10 x 15 inch rectangle. Top with strawberries and chocolate chips.
4. Put in the freezer until firm. This usually takes 3 hours,
5. Cut into 32 pieces. Enjoy!

*Cheesy Brussels Sprouts Chips*

Servings: 4

Ingredients:

- 15 Brussels sprouts
- 1 teaspoon yeast
- 1 tablespoon olive oil
- ⅛ teaspoon salt (or to taste)
- ¼ teaspoon ground pepper (or to taste)
- 2 tablespoons shredded parmesan cheese

Instructions:

1. Preheat your oven to 400°F.

2. Remove outer leaves from Brussels sprouts and transfer to a large bowl until you have enough to make about 4 cups. Add the olive oil and seasoning. Gentle massage with clean hands to allow leaves to absorb flavor.

3. Place as one layer on a baking sheet.

4. Roast leaves until browned and crispy, which should take about 10 minutes. Sprinkle with Parmesan cheese.

*Oat-Peanut Butter Balls*

Servings:12


Ingredients:

- ½ cup rolled oats
- ¾ cup chopped Medjool dates (you may also use raisins or dried cranberries)
- ¼ cup natural peanut butter


Instructions:

1. Fill small bowl with hot water, and soak Medjool dates for about 10 minutes, and then drain.
2. Place all ingredients in a food processor. Process until all

ingredients are very finely chopped.

3. Roll into 12 balls. Put in the fridge for at least 15 minutes. This snack can keep for up to a week.

*Week 2*

You probably got used to eating healthier foods by now. By this time, your body has probably adjusted to the lower calorie intake for the past week. You won't be craving as much food especially since the technique we recommended does not ask you to deprive yourself.

Still, for weeks 2 to 4, we'll take it up a notch. From limiting your consumption to 1500, you could go further down to around 1200 calories per day. That is still within the healthy weight loss threshold if your recommended daily intake (without a weight loss target) used to be 2000.

For week 2, you can try some of the recipes mentioned in the meal plan for your first week. You can also try the following meal ideas. You are free to try other recipes and experiment as you'd like so long as you look up the calorie count.

*Monday*

- Berry smoothie (½ of a banana, a cup of frozen strawberries, half cup of plain, low-fat Greek yogurt, and half cup nonfat milk)
- 2 cups of vegetable soup
- 4 ounces of grilled chicken, half cup of sweet potatoes (roasted), and a cup of frozen Brussels sprouts

Total Calories: 1230

*Tuesday*

- Oats with blueberries (Half cup of oats mix in a tablespoon of chia seeds, half cup of nonfat milk, 1/2 cup of plain and low-fat Greek yogurt, and 1/2 cup of blueberries)
- Salad made of 3 ounces of tuna, 2 cups of mixed greens, a cup of cherry tomatoes, chopped cucumber, and 1 tablespoon of vinaigrette.
- Plated meal with 4 ounces of grilled chicken, ½ cup of roasted sweet potatoes, and a cup of roasted Brussels sprouts

Total Calories: 1303

*Wednesday*

- 2 slices of whole-wheat toast and 2 hard boiled eggs. You can add hot sauce if you want to
- 3 ounces of smoked salmon, 1/4 of an avocado, and a cup of mixed greens wrapped in a whole-wheat tortilla
- A plate with 4 ounces of pan-fried lean steak, a cup of roasted sweet potatoes, and a 1 cup of roasted Brussels sprouts

Total Calories: 1358


*Thursday*

- Breakfast tortilla made with 1 scrambled egg and 1/2 cup of

black beans. Wrap it with a piece of whole wheat tortilla
- Sandwich made of 2 whole wheat bread slices, 3 ounces of lean turkey, a cup of mixed greens, and 1/4 of an avocado
- 2 slices of a veggie pizza and a cup of salad greens

Total Calories: 1306


*Friday*

- Green smoothie made with half of a banana, half of a small avocado, half cup of non-fat milk, half cup of low-fat Greek yogurt, 1/2 cup of frozen mango, and 1 cup of kale
- 2 cups of vegetable soup

- Plate of 4 ounces salmon, 1 cup each of steamed carrots and broccoli, a teaspoon of sesame seeds, and 2 tablespoons of teriyaki sauce

Total Calories: 1226


*Saturday*

- Same breakfast as Tuesday
- Tortilla wrap made of a whole wheat tortilla, a cup of mixed greens, 1/4 of an avocado, and 3 ounces of lean turkey
- Dinner plate with 4 ounces of shrimp, one cup each for both broccoli and carrots, half cup of brown rice (cooked), and 2 tablespoons of teriyaki sauce

Total Calories: 1383


*Sunday*

- Green smoothie (same as Friday)
- Lunch plate made of 3 ounces grilled chicken, one cup each of cucumber and cherry tomatoes, 1/2 cup of cooked quinoa, 2 tablespoons of feta cheese, and a tablespoon of vinaigrette
- Dinner plate made of 4 ounces mahi-mahi, one cup each of both steamed broccoli and carrots, a tablespoon of sesame seeds, and 2 tablespoons of teriyaki sauce

Total Calories: 1239 calories

In this meal plan, the mix and match is clear. For some days, we can see the same ingredients are used to make food. The only differences are the protein source. You can adapt this same idea in making your own meals.

As for intermittent fasting, you can start implementing it now. With your reduced calorie intake, we recommend that you start with a 14 hour fast and 10 hour period.

For example, you can implement an 8 AM to 6 PM eating period. That way, you still get all your meals and have enough time for fasting. The addition of fasting will make you lose more weight and combats plateau.

*Weeks 3 and 4*

We'll continue with the trend of consuming just 1200 calories for the remaining 2 weeks of the month. After all, you got used to this calorie limit already for the past week.

This can be your diet plan for the remaining weeks. Feel free to change it depending on how your preference and available ingredients.

Day 1

- A combination of 3/4 cup of bran flakes, a piece of banana, and a cup of fat-free milk in a bowl
- Sandwich using a small-sized whole pita bread, 3 ounces of

turkey breast, a teaspoon of mayonnaise, mustard, 1/2 of a whole roasted pepper, and lettuce
- 4 ounces of broiled flounder, 2 pieces of sliced plum tomatoes, a cup of cooked couscous, and 1 cup of steamed broccoli. Sprinkle with grated Parmesan cheese.

Day 2

- Smoothie made of a cup of frozen berries, 1/2 of a banana, and 8 ounces of fat-free milk. Take 1 or 2 pieces of hard-boiled eggs for the road
- A cup of vegetable soup, a cup of grapes, and vegetable burger wrapped in whole grain pita

- 4 ounces of grilled, boneless, and skinless chicken breast, and 1/2 piece of baked or plain sweet potato

Day 3

- 1/2 cup of quick-cook oatmeal with unsweetened or low-fat soy milk. Add 1/2 of sliced apples, a teaspoon of honey, and a pinch of cinnamon
- Chicken salad with sliced red grapes, a tablespoon of light mayonnaise, and 1 tablespoon of unsweetened Greek yogurt
- 4 ounces of steamed shrimp and 1 baked potato, 3 cups of steamed spinach, and a tablespoon of Greek yogurt

Day 4

- Half of a toasted English muffin, half of a small apple, and 2/3 cup of plain and unsweetened Greek yogurt
- A cup of tomato soup and sandwich made in a small whole wheat pita and 3 ounces of sliced roast beef, a teaspoon of horseradish, tomato slices, mustard, and lettuce.
- 3 ounces of poached salmon paired with 3/4 cup of quinoa and apple.

Day 5

- A cup of Cheerios mixed with a tablespoon of slivered almonds,

1/2 cup of berries, and 6 ounces of plain and unsweetened Greek yogurt

- Quesadilla with 1/4 cup of refried beans, 1/2 cup of low-fat cottage cheese, cucumber spears, and clementines
- 3 ounces of roasted pork tenderloin, a cup of baked acorn squash, and 2 to 3 cups of greens.


Day 6

- Toast a whole-grain frozen waffle and serve it with 2 tablespoons of nut butter, a piece of a small-sized banana, nutmeg, and cinnamon

- Tuna pita with cucumber and onion slices, a tablespoon of light mayo, and mustard
- Jambalaya and 3 cups of spinach sauteed in a tablespoon of olive oil with garlic

Day 7

- English muffin with a tomato slice, poached egg, and 1/2 cup of steamed spinach
- Black bean salad that includes 1/2 cup of mandarin orange, red onion, scallions, chopped red bell pepper, and stone ground corn tortilla
- 3 ounces of broiled flank steak, a piece of baked sweet potato, a cup

of steamed zucchini, and 1 1/2
cup of berries


Day 8

- Greek yogurt with honey and
  blueberries
- Whole wheat toast with avocado
  and white bean
- A cup of balsamic roasted
  cauliflower with Parmesan cheese
  and a serving of creamy chicken
  and mushrooms


Day 9

- A piece of hard-boiled egg and a
  teaspoon of hot sauce

- A serving of apple and cheddar in a pita pocket
- A serving of sweet potato stuffed with black beans and hummus dressing

## Day 10

- Peanut butter and banana toast
- 4 cups of salad made with figs and goat cheese
- 3/4 cup of cooked quinoa and a serving of poached salmon and asparagus

## Day 11

- Greek yogurt with fruits and nuts

- A bowl of black bean quinoa with hummus dressing
- 5 ounces of cooked chicken breast and winter salad with balsamic berry vinaigrette

Day 12

- Greek yogurt with honey and blueberries (mix in 1 1/2 tablespoons of almonds for a different taste
- Green salad with hummus and pita bread
- A serving of roasted root vegetables with polenta and goat cheese

Day 13

- Cooked rolled oats with raspberries, cinnamon, and maple syrup
- A serving of veggies and quinoa salad
- 3 and 1/2 cup of vegetable soup

Day 14

- 2 and 1/2 cups of baby kale salad with egg and bacon
- 2 cups of vegetable soup
- A serving of vegetable and chicken pita, and garlic mayo

As you can see for the 3rd and 4th week, we recommended simple recipes. This is because we'd like to show you a sustainable way to prepare food that promote weight loss. There is a way to enjoy healthy food and it does not take a lot of ingredients or preparation time.

If you want to try intermittent fasting, you can go for the 16:8 method at this point. You can still eat all meals by having breakfast at a later time. Since you're eating a lot less than before, you can afford to just have a small gap in-between breakfast and lunch (say, 10 AM for breakfast and 12 noon or 1 PM for lunch). You can also choose to cut off one of your meals, either you skip breakfast or dinner. Also, there's a shorter gap between breakfast and lunch than it is between lunch and dinner.

# Conclusion

We hope that this book has been of some help to you.

In weight loss, winning the mental battle means winning half the battle. That's why it's important that you make dieting an enjoyable part of your life – not as a punishment.

The recipes included in this book are delicious and healthy that you won't feel like you're missing out on anything. We also hope that the small tips on Chapter 2 would help you get into the right mindset so that if you do lapse every once in a while, you remain kind to yourself and able to steer yourself to the right track.

Eating is a huge part of any weight loss regimen. Knowing what to eat and, hopefully seeing patterns as to which foods should be consumed is a great way to lose weight – and to keep the weight off.

Weight gain doesn't happen overnight. But it doesn't have to be a punishment that you'd have to bear for the rest of your life. It also doesn't mean that it takes a lifetime to reverse the ravages of excess weight. You can see the difference in just 30 days, if you start now.

We hope that this ebook will help you get to that difference, and keep going well after.